How To Lose Weight Without Dieting For A Day

Action Plan To Lose Weight While Eating What You Like

Jessica Mace

Text Copyright © Jessica Mace

Legal & Disclaimer

The information contained in this book and its contents is not designed to replace or take the place of any form of medical or professional advice; and is not meant to replace the need for independent medical, financial, legal or other professional advice or services, as may be required. The content and information in this book has been provided for educational and entertainment purposes only.

The content and information contained in this book has been compiled from sources deemed reliable, and it is accurate to the best of the Author's knowledge, information and belief. However, the Author cannot guarantee its accuracy and validity and cannot be held liable for any errors and/or omissions. Further, changes are periodically made to this book as and when needed. Where appropriate and/or necessary, you must consult a professional (including but not limited to your doctor, attorney, financial advisor or such other professional advisor) before using any of the suggested remedies, techniques, or information in this book.

Upon using the contents and information contained in this book, you agree to hold harmless the Author from and against any damages, costs, and expenses, including any legal fees potentially resulting from the application of any of the information provided by this book. This disclaimer applies to any loss, damages or injury caused by the use and application, whether directly or indirectly, of any advice or information presented, whether for breach of contract, tort, negligence, personal injury, criminal intent, or under any other cause of action.

You agree to accept all risks of using the information presented inside this book.

You agree that by continuing to read this book, where appropriate and/or necessary, you shall consult a professional (including but not limited to your doctor, attorney, or financial advisor or such other advisor as needed) before using any of the suggested remedies, techniques, or information in this book.

INTRODUCTION

Obesity is epidemic in the United States. The number of overweight and obese Americans has grown at a disturbing rate, especially over the past few years, to the point where today more Americans are overweight than are normal weight. In fact, over sixty percent of Americans are now considered to be overweight, with over 30 percent of the population considered to be obese (e.g., overweight by more than 20-30% of recommended weight). These numbers describe a tragic public health situation. Being overweight increases a person's risk of serious illness. A very large (and growing) percentage of citizens are at increased risk for developing serious chronic diseases, and face the prospect of early disability or death as the result of being overweight. Meanwhile, the entire society struggles under the burden of the resulting increase in health care costs.

This book concerns weight loss, an issue perpetually on many people's minds. Almost everyone wants to be slim and toned, but the reality is that it is far easier to gain weight than to lose it. In the following pages, causes of weight gain are reviewed, along with numerous reasons why people should devote the effort necessary to reduce their weight to recommended levels. Having provided motivation for a weight loss program, I conclude with weight loss methods, and suggestions for achieving permanent healthy weight loss. Get started now by turning the page.

Jessica Mace

CHAPTER ONE

WHY DOES WEIGHT MATTER?

People come in all shapes and sizes and what might be a healthy weight for one person isn't necessarily healthy for another. It's not healthy to be too thin or to carry too much body fat – you need to find the weight that's best for you by checking with your doctor, and then trying to achieve and maintain it.

The problem with carrying too much body fat (medically referred to as being overweight) is that it can increase your risk of a number of health problems. These include:

- Coronary heart disease

- Diabetes

- High blood pressure

- High cholesterol

- Gall bladder disease

- Joint problems, e.g. gout, arthritis and joint pain

- Sleep problems, e.g. sleep apnoea

- Certain types of cancer.

Your risk of developing these health conditions depends not just on your weight, but also on other risk factors that you may have.

WHY DO WE PUT ON WEIGHT?

Body weight is affected by a number of factors, but the two key factors are:

1. The amount of energy (kilojoules) that we put into our bodies from food and drinks

2. The amount of energy (kilojoules) that we use up through physical activity and other daily activities.

Put simply, it's all about what goes in and what gets used up.

People often get confused by energy and kilojoules – energy and kilojoules are the same thing. Kilojoules are just a measure of energy, in the same way as centimeters or inches are a measure of length. Energy is like fuel in a car – it's what keeps us moving and able to go about our daily activities.

You will gain weight if:

1. You eat and drink more than your body needs – you take in too much energy (kilojoules)

2. You aren't active enough – you don't use up enough energy (kilojoules)

3. If you do both – you eat and drink too much and are not active enough.

Achieving a healthy weight is a real balancing act. It works like this:

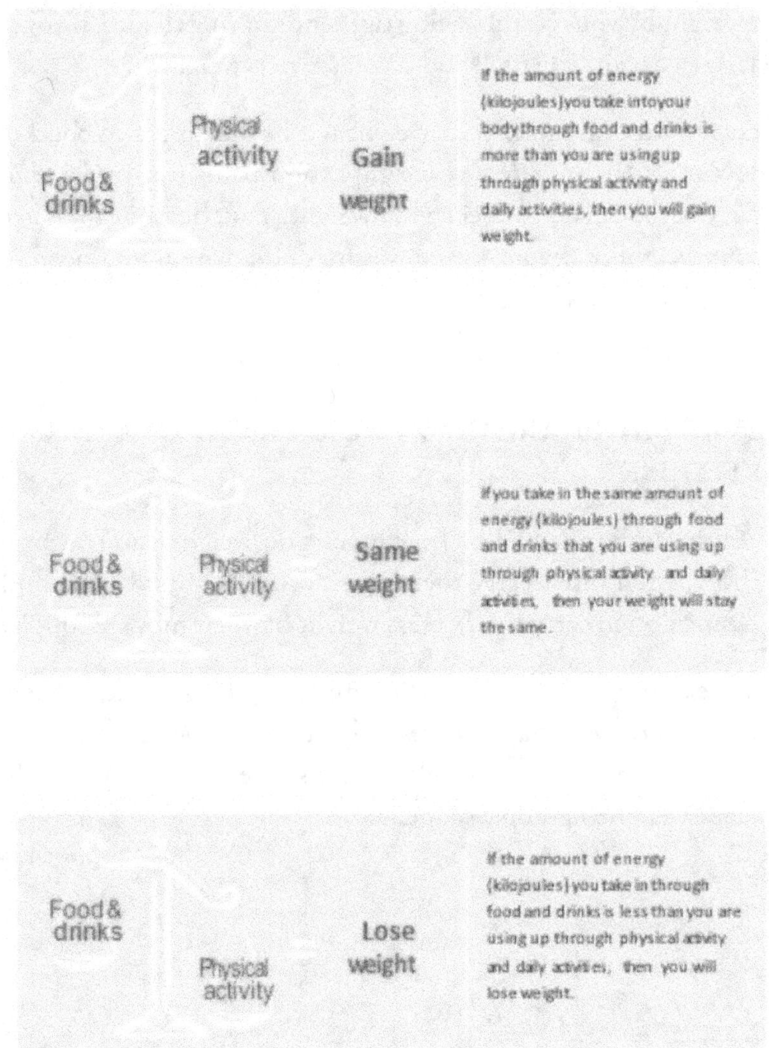

IS MY WEIGHT A HEALTH RISK?

Some people think they are overweight when they aren't; others think their weight is fine when it isn't. While you can generally tell if you've put on weight by your clothes being tighter or having to loosen your belt a notch or two, this won't tell you if you are overweight.

The best way to find out if your weight is a health risk is to check with your doctor. There are a few very simple and pain- free measurements that your doctor can do to check your weight. Your doctor can then consider your weight and your overall health and advise if you need to do something about your weight.

EXCESS WEIGHT AROUND YOUR MIDDLE IS A GREATER HEALTH RISK

Your health can be affected by how much you weigh as well as by your body shape. Men often carry their excess weight around their middle, while women often carry their excess weight on their hips and thighs.

Carrying excess weight around your middle (being 'apple shaped') is more of a health risk than if excess weight is on your hips and thighs (being 'pear shaped'). The so-called 'pear shape' is actually a healthier body shape than being 'apple shaped'.

CHAPTER TWO

IF I NEED TO LOSE WEIGHT, WHAT DO I DO?

If your weight is a health risk or is affecting your enjoyment of life, you need to do something about it. To lose weight, you need to use up more energy (kilojoules) than you are taking in. This means that you need to look at how you can reduce your energy (kilojoule) intake and increase your energy (kilojoule) output. That all comes down to the food and drinks you consume – what types and how much – and the type and amount of physical activity you do.

Despite what various books and diets may say, losing weight in a healthy way is not quick and it's not simple. Fad or crash diets are often unhealthy and are not helpful with losing weight and keeping it off in the longer term. People have generally put their weight on over a period of time, maybe even years, so it's not going to come off overnight. What can change overnight though is your commitment to make some changes to your eating patterns, to increase your physical activity levels, and to reduce the amount of time you spend sitting.

Once you've decided to make a change, you need to work out your plan. This plan will help you to work out where you can make changes, what changes you will make and to be realistic about what you can achieve.

STEP 1

SET REALISTIC WEIGHT LOSS OR LIFESTYLE GOALS

Set yourself realistic goals. It may just be one goal or you might set a couple at the same time. The key is to choose a goal or goals that suit you. This will help to keep you motivated and stop you trying to do too much too soon. For example, some realistic goals might be:

• To stop gaining weight – if you have recently been gaining weight, this is a useful goal to start with

• To lose 2 kg in the next two months – this may not sound like much and may sound very slow, but if you can do this and keep this weight off, then that is a fantastic effort.

If you make your goal too difficult, you can end up feeling like a failure when it really isn't your fault. For example:

• To lose 10 kg in 10 weeks – this is not easy. Losing 10 kg may take months to achieve, possibly 12 months or more, if you are losing weight healthily.

It's much better to choose small goals and lose weight gradually than set a goal that seems unachievable. Even if you only ever lose a few kilograms, it can make a big difference to your health, and it's better than continuing to gain weight.

Your goals can focus on a change in weight, but they could also focus on changing your eating patterns, increasing your physical activity levels and reducing your sitting time. For example, some goals might be:

• To limit the number of times you buy take-out foods to once a week

• To go for a 30 minute walk on at least three evenings each week

• To reduce the amount of TV you watch each day.

Try not to become 'ruled' by the scales. If you want to weigh yourself, make sure it's no more than once a week. Always remember that the amount of weight you lose is only one way of measuring your achievements.

Some other important ways to measure how well you are doing include:

- How you feel

- If your clothes are looser

- If you can do things without getting tired.

And if you've managed to improve your eating patterns, increase the amount of physical activity you do, and reduce the amount of time you spend sitting each day, that's positive for your overall health even if you don't manage to lose any weight.

CHAPTER THREE

STEP 2

IDENTIFY WHAT YOU EAT AND DRINK, YOUR LEVEL OF PHYSICAL ACTIVITY AND AMOUNT OF SITTING TIME

To do this, you might like to keep a diary for a week. Keeping a diary can help you to see where you can make changes.

If keeping a diary works for you, here are some tips on how to do it.

TIPS ON KEEPING A FOOD AND DRINKS DIARY

• Using a notebook, notepad or computer, write down everything you eat and drink each day.

• If you can, also include the amount of food or drinks you have.

• Don't forget to write down snacks as well.

• Write down the time of eating/drinking and where you were eating/drinking, such as at home with the family, on my own in front of the TV or at a café.

TIPS ON KEEPING A PHYSICAL ACTIVITY AND SITTING DIARY

• Use your computer or the same notebook or notepad that you use for your food diary, or use a separate one.

• Write down all the times you are active – write what you do, what part of the day you are being active and for how long, including: any planned activity you do, such as going to the gym, jogging or playing sport, activity, such as housework, gardening, taking the stairs instead of a lift, walking to the local shops, walking the dog.

• Believe it or not, it's also very useful to record the amount of time you spend sitting. Write down what it is you are doing when you are sitting, such as watching TV, working or driving the car.

Recording both your active and sitting time will help you to work out how active or inactive you are, the times you are active and inactive, and where you could try to make changes to increase your physical activity levels and reduce your sitting time.

CHAPTER FOUR

STEP 3

MAKE CHANGES TO WHAT YOU EAT AND DRINK

If you've kept a food and drinks diary, use the information from your diary with the following information to help to identify changes you can make.

Healthy eating for weight loss is about making sure you are still getting all the nutrients you need for good health while reducing the amount of energy (kilojoules) you take in.

The good news is that many foods that are lower in energy (kilojoules) are also packed full of nutrients –and these are the types of foods you need to eat most.

CHOOSE FOODS AND DRINKS LOWER IN ENERGY (KILO-JOULES)

FOODS

Vegetables, fruit and legumes (for example, split peas, kidney beans, baked beans, three bean mix, lentils and chickpeas) provide some energy (kilojoules) but they are also packed full of vitamins, minerals and fiber. Eating these sorts of foods helps to make you feel full, without giving you too much energy (kilojoules).

Other lower energy (kilojoule) food choices that also provide a range of vitamins and minerals include:

• Reduced, low or no fat milk and yoghurt.

• Lean meat and poultry (meat trimmed of all visible fat and chicken without skin) and fish.

• Wholegrain or whole meal bread and breakfast cereals, plain pasta (preferably whole meal), plain rice (preferably brown) and plain noodles.

• Including all of these types of foods in your daily eating plan will help to ensure you are getting all the nutrients you need without a lot of extra energy (kilojoules).

DRINKS

Plain water is by far the best option because it has no energy (kilojoules). It's also cheap and quenches your thirst.

Other suitable choices to include in moderation are plain mineral water; soda water; reduced, low or no fat milk; herbal tea; and tea or coffee (if you have milk, use reduced, low or no fat varieties or 'added calcium' soy milk).

LIMIT HIGH ENERGY (KILOJOULE) FOODS AND DRINKS

The types of foods and drinks that often contain lots of energy (kilojoules) are listed below.

FOODS

• Chocolate, confectionery

• Potato crisps and other savory snack foods, such as corn crisps

• Cakes, sweet biscuits

• Pastries – sweet and savory

• Take-away foods, such as deep-fried foods, creamy pasta dishes, cheesy dishes and hamburgers.

DRINKS

• Soft drinks, fruit juices, fruit juice drinks, cordials and alcoholic drinks.

You can still have these types of foods and drinks occasionally, but they really do provide a lot of energy (kilojoules) without giving you much else. Try to only have these types of foods and drinks as a treat or for a special occasion. Eating them daily or regularly throughout the week would lead to weight gain for most people. Take a look at the tables on the pages below to see just how much energy (kilojoules) you could save by having a lower energy (kilojoule) food or drink choice, rather than a high energy (kilojoule) food or drink choice.

WATCH YOUR OVERALL FOOD AND DRINK INTAKE

It is easy to eat more than your body needs, so be aware of the amount of food and drinks (other than water) you are having. This isn't about starving yourself, skipping meals or going thirsty. It's about eating when you actually feel hungry rather than eating because of the clock or just because food is there.

If you feel hungry all the time or find yourself wanting to eat all the time, you probably need to visit your doctor and seek some guidance about why this may be the case. Your doctor may refer you to another health professional, such as an accredited practicing dietitian, for specific advice.

When eating out or buying take-away food, be careful about how much food you order. In many cases, you can buy a large meal or a meal pack for around the same price as a smaller meal or an individual item. The trap here is that you end up eating a larger serving or more food than you actually need.

Try to limit your intake of high energy (kilojoule) drinks, such as alcohol, soft drinks, fruit juices and cordials. Make plain water your main drink choice and drink plenty of this throughout the day to make sure you don't go thirsty. Only have high energy (kilojoule) drinks occasionally and limit the amount.

CAN I HAVE ALCOHOL?

Alcohol is high in energy (kilojoules). Often when drinking alcohol, we tend to also snack on high energy (kilojoule) foods, such as potato or corn crisps, pastries and nuts.

You can still enjoy alcohol while trying to lose weight, you just have to limit how much you have.

TIPS TO LOWER YOUR ALCOHOL INTAKE

• Drink water or plain mineral water first to quench your thirst, then have an alcoholic drink.

• Alternate a glass of alcohol with a low energy (kilojoule) drink, such as water or plain mineral water.

• Where appropriate, mix your alcoholic drink with plain mineral water, soda or diet soft drink.

• Use only half-measures of spirits.

• Choose a low alcohol or light beer.

• Choose a low alcohol wine if available.

• Always have water available at the table, whether you are dining out or at home.

• Use diet soft drinks in mixed drinks, for example diet cola with rum, or diet ginger ale with brandy.

• Take your time with each drink.

- Use smaller glasses.

MODIFYING RECIPES

Many of your favorite recipes need only simple changes to reduce their energy (kilojoules) or their saturated fat content. The two steps to changing a recipe are:

1. Try healthier cooking methods

2. Change ingredients by reducing, removing or replacing with something else.

METHOD HEALTHIER COOKING METHOD

Deep-fry
Roast in the oven on a lined tray or grill tray. Food can be lightly steamed or microwaved first, then brushed with oil such as canola, sunflower, soybean or olive oil for crispness. Crumbed fish, chicken and oven fries can be cooked in the oven rather than deep-fried.

Shallow-fry/Sauté
Stir-fry using reduced salt stock and/or oil, such as canola, sunflower, soybean, olive or peanut oil. Try using a non-stick fry pan.

Roast
Choose lean cuts of meat or trim all visible fat and then place the meat on a rack in a baking dish with 1 to 2 cm water. For extra flavour, add herbs to the water. Try brushing with a marinade to prevent the meat drying out, or cover the food with a lid or aluminium foil for part of the cooking time. Roasting on a spit or rotisserie will allow fat to drip away. Brush or spray vegetables with oil such as canola, sunflower, soybean, olive or peanut oil, and bake in a separate pan.

Casserole/Stew
Trim fat off meat before cooking. Add legumes, such as kidney beans, chickpeas, soy beans or lentils, for extra fibre and flavour. After cooking, chill the food so any fat solidifies on the surface. Skim the fat off the surface before reheating and thickening (if necessary).

INGREDIENT HEALTHIER ALTERNATIVE

Milk/Yoghurt/ Cream

Use reduced, low or no fat varieties. Use ricotta cheese whipped with a little icing sugar, fruit or reduced, low or no fat milk as a substitute for cream.

Sour cream

Blend cottage cheese and reduced, low or no fat milk (add a little lemon juice or vinegar if desired). Use reduced, low or no fat natural yoghurt. Use evaporated reduced fat milk and lemon juice.

Cheese

Use smaller amounts of reduced fat varieties. Use a little grated parmesan cheese instead of grated cheddar – it gives more flavor and less is needed. Mix grated reduced fat cheese with oats, breadcrumbs or wheat germ for toppings on casseroles, gratins and baked dishes.

Butter/ Margarine spreads

Use margarine spreads made from canola, sunflower or olive oil, and dairy blends that have earned the Heart Foundation Tick instead of butter, other dairy blends, lard, copha or cooking fats. Note: reduced fat or 'lite' spreads are generally not good for cooking.

Oil

Use a variety of oils for cooking. Some suitable choices include canola, sunflower, soybean, olive and peanut oil.

Mayonnaise/ Dressing

Use salad dressings and mayonnaise made from oils such as canola, sunflower, soybean and olive oil. Make your own using ingredients such as reduced, low or no fat yoghurt, buttermilk, tomato paste, balsamic or other vinegars, lemon juice, ricotta cheese, mustard and fruit pulp.

Meat/Poultry

Choose lean meats and poultry. Remove all visible fat from meat and skin from poultry before cooking. Marinate or add flavor with ingredients such as wine

	vinegars. Sear meat quickly to keep in juices.
	Use margarine spreads made from canola, sunflower or olive oil, or dairy blends that have earned the Heart Foundation Tick instead of butter. Use oils such as canola, sunflower or olive oil. The minimum
Cakes/Biscuits	fat required for biscuits is about 2 tablespoons per cup of flour – this will retain crispness. Make plain sponges, yeast cakes, breads, muffins and scones as they generally use less fat. Use wholegrain or whole meal flour to add some extra fiber.
Pastry/Savoury	Use filo pastry, brushing every three to four layers with oil such as canola, sunflower, soybean or olive oil, egg white or reduced, low or no fat yoghurt. Use pastry made with oil such as canola, sunflower or olive oil.
Coconut cream/Coconut Milk	Use evaporated reduced fat milk with a little coconut essence. Alternatively, if you have time, soak desiccated coconut in warm reduced, low or no fat milk for 30 minutes, then strain, discard the coconut and use the milk. For occasional use, try a reduced fat coconut milk.

COMPARISON OF ENERGY (KILOJOULE) CONTENT OF FOODS AND DRINKS

Here are some examples of how you can make small but important changes to your eating habits. Remember it's the small changes that can make a big difference!

Also remember that these are just examples. The key is to think about what changes you could make in your food choices and the way you prepare and cook foods that will help to lower energy (kilojoules).

LESS HEALTHY FOOD CHOICES	KJ CONTENT	HEALTHIER FOOD CHOICES	KJ CONTENT
1 plain large croissant (70 g) with 2 tsp butter and 2 tsp jam	1600	2 pieces wholemeal plain toast (30 g each) with 1 tsp margarine spread and 1 tsp jam per slice	970
2 breakfast wheat biscuits (30 g) + 2/3 cup full fat milk	887	2 breakfast wheat biscuits (30 g) + 2/3 cup skim milk	756
1 plain donut (70 g)	1045	1 medium banana (150 g)	365
1 packet potato crisps (50 g)	1045	1 medium apple (150 g)	270
2 choc-coated cream biscuits	743	2 plain sweet biscuits	277
1 chocolate bar (50 g)	1110	Small handful of almonds (~ 20) 20 g	473
1 meat pie (175 g)	1880	Ham and salad sandwich (made with 2 tsp margarine)	1105
Hungarian salami (30 g)	535	Ham, plain fresh (30 g)	174
1 cappuccino (1 cup) with full cream milk	375	1 cappuccino (1 cup) with skim milk	210
1 glass cola soft drink (250 mL)	440	1 glass low sugar or diet cola soft drink	4
Orange juice	400	1 glass water	0

(sweetened) (250 mL)			
1 glass dry white wine (100 mL)	263	1 glass dry white wine – reduced alcohol (100 mL)	167
1 stubbie/can full strength beer	585	1 stubbie/can light beer	260
Pan-fried chicken parmigiana	2050	Pan-fried chicken breast, no skin (100 g)	795
1 medium T-bone steak with fat, grilled	1255	1 medium T-bone steak, trimmed of visible fat, grilled	960
Hamburger mince, 25% fat (100 g)	1230	Lean mince, 10% fat (100 g)	710
Chicken breast with skin, roasted without added fat (100 g)	920	Chicken breast, without skin, roasted without added fat (100 g)	605
1 fillet white fish, e.g. whiting, fried in batter (150 g)	1725	1 fillet white fish, e.g. whiting, steamed, poached or grilled (150 g)	630

WHAT TO LOOK FOR ON A FOOD LABEL TO FIND ENERGY (KILOJOULES)

By law, all food labels in Australia must contain a nutrition information panel and an ingredients list. The only exceptions to this are foods that are sold in very small packages, herbs, spices, tea, coffee and food made and packaged at the point of sale, although some food outlets do provide this information.

The nutrition information panel is where you will find information about how much energy (kilojoules) the food or drink contains.

This will tell you how much energy (kilojoules) there is in 100 g or 100 mL and in each serving of the food or drink. You can use this when comparing similar products to help you to choose the one lower in energy (kilojoules). For example, if you were comparing two types of sweet biscuits, you would choose the one that provided the least amount of energy (kilojoules) in 100 g.

The ingredient listing on the label can also help you to identify whether or not the food is high in energy (kilojoules). Ingredients are listed in order by weight. The main ingredient by weight will be listed first and the smallest listed last. If the first few ingredients in the ingredients list are high in fat and/ or sugar, then the food/drink is likely to be high in energy (kilojoules). Some examples of ingredients that are high in fat and sugar are listed in the table below.

High-fat, high-sugar ingredients

Fat		Sugar	
Vegetable oil	Coconut oil	Sucrose	Glucose syrup
Vegetable fat	Palm oil	Maltose	Corn syrup Golden
Animal fat	Chocolate chips	Lactose	syrup
Animal oil	Milk solids	Dextrose	Disaccharides
Shortening	Monoglycerides	Fructose	Monosaccharides
		Glucose	Polysaccharides
		Molasses	Honey
		Malt extract	

Note the words 'creamed', 'toasted', 'mayonnaise' can also indicate added fat. [illegible]

CHAPTER FIVE

STEP 4

INCREASE YOUR PHYSICAL ACTIVITY LEVELS AND REDUCE YOUR SITTING TIME

If you've kept a physical activity and sitting diary, use the information from your diary together with the following information to help to identify how you can be more physically active and reduce the time you spend sitting.

Being physically active uses up energy (kilojoules). The more you move, the more energy (kilojoules) you will burn. So think about movement as an opportunity to improve your health, rather than a time-wasting inconvenience.

HOW MUCH ACTIVITY DO I NEED TO DO?

Thirty minutes of physical activity on most or all days of the week is great for your general health and well-being, regardless of your body weight or shape. For some people, this may even be enough to prevent weight gain.

If you need to lose weight or are gaining weight, then you will need to do more than the 30 minutes of physical activity each day recommended for general health.

The bottom line is that you need to increase your physical activity levels and reduce the amount of time that you spend sitting, so focus on these things first. Gradually, try to build up the amount of time you are physically active and reduce the amount of time you spend sitting. Don't worry about how active other people are, just focus on trying to increase your own activity level.

If you can enjoy some vigorous activity as well, then that's even better. Vigorous activity, such as doing a gym class, playing sport or jogging, gives additional health, fitness and weight loss benefits.

It's all about you – the amount of activity that will work for you is likely to be different to what will work for someone else.

Just as some people seem to be able to eat and drink whatever they like without putting on weight, some people may also seem to be able to get away with doing little, if any, activity to keep their weight down. That doesn't matter. What matters is what is right and comfortable for you. So get active today!

GETTING PHYSICALLY ACTIVE

There are really three ways to get active.

1. FIT IT INTO YOUR DAY

The easiest way is to think about how to make physical activity a part of your day – that is, how can you be active while doing something else that has to be done anyway? Think about how you can be physically active in as many ways as you can. Even though our lives are very busy, there are lots of ways to fit physical activity into our daily routine. Some of the following ideas may help to get you started.

AT HOME

- Get off the couch and change the TV channels instead of using the remote.

- Get off the couch or off the chair – the more you sit on it, the less active you will be.

- Walk into the next room to speak to a family member rather than shouting through walls.

• Watch one less TV program each week and instead do something active during that time – go walking, do some housework or gardening, play games with the kids.

• If you have a garden, tend to it yourself – weeding, planting, digging, mowing the lawn will all help to burn off extra kilos and it can be fun at the same time.

• Housework – ironing, vacuuming, dusting, hand washing clothes, polishing furniture – may not seem like fun, but it burns up energy and somebody has to do it.

• Wash the car by hand – it's good for you and for saving water.

• Walk the dog if you have one – it's great for both of you.

• Clean out the cupboards, storage areas, garage or shed.

• Wash the windows – inside and out.

• Walk to the letterbox to post letters rather than waiting until the next time you're out in the car.

• Get a cordless phone and walk around while using it, rather than sitting down.

AT WORK

• Visit your colleague in their workspace instead of phoning or sending an email.

• Take a break or use your lunch break to go for a walk – even 10 to 15 minutes is a good effort. Ask some others to go with you.

• If there are stairs, use them.

- If you sit at a desk all day in front of a computer, do some stretching exercises at least once a day.

- Try to get away from your desk throughout the day.

- Do some filing.

GOING PLACES

- Walk, ride your bike or rollerblade instead of driving.

- If you can't do it all the way, at least do it part of the way.

- Forget about finding the closest parking space – park further away and just walk the extra distance.

- Get off the bus/tram/train one or two stops earlier and

- Count to 10 before jumping in the car – just think about whether you really need to drive or not. The less you drive the car, the better it is for you and for the environment.

SOCIAL

- Catch up with friends for a walk.

- Go on outings that encourage you to walk around, such as visiting the zoo, gardens, fun parks, expos or historic sites.

- Visit the local park and take a picnic.

- Arrange to do active things with friends, such as bowling (ten pin or lawn), sailing, bike riding, tennis, rock climbing, dancing (all types), swimming or bushwalking.

- Join a local community walking group or try something new, such as belly dancing, tai chi or yoga.

2. DO SOME PLANNED PHYSICAL ACTIVITY

The second way to get more active and burn off extra kilos is to try to set aside some time each day for planned physical activity.

Many people struggle with this, saying that they don't have time to be physically active. And it is hard to find time when you have lots of other priorities, such as work, family commitments and social functions. It's really about making physical activity a priority for you. Try to get some planned activity into your life at least three times a week. Then try to build that up over time.

WHAT ARE SOME EXAMPLES OF PLANNED PHYSICAL ACTIVITY?

Doing any of the following sorts of activities on a regular basis for a set amount of time is planned physical activity:

• Go for a walk or a jog

• Go to a gym class – weights, aerobics, spin or pump

• Play a sport – cricket, netball, football, volleyball, rugby, soccer, badminton, squash, tennis or volleyball

• Go for a swim

• Do yoga, tai chi or pilates.

If some of your planned physical activity is vigorous activity – that is, it makes you really breathe hard and sweat – then it will bring extra health, fitness and weight loss benefits.

Using a pedometer is a great motivator for helping to increase your physical activity levels.

Pedometers are small instruments that clip onto your clothing and measure how much walking or running you are doing. Some will also tell you how much energy (kilojoules) you have burned.

3. SIT LESS

If you are sitting down then you are generally not being active – chair activity classes are an exception to this.

If you've been recording in a diary how much time in a day you spend sitting down, you'll have a good idea of where you could make some changes. Always think about whether there is a way that you can be physically active rather than sitting down – then do it!

I'M ALREADY ACTIVE – WHAT CAN I DO?

If you are already active, but are putting on weight or are overweight, then you still need to think about how you can be more active. You also need to look at your eating habits and see if there are any changes you need to make.

Review what you are doing and see if you can include more planned physical activity sessions or if there are other ways that you could build more activity into your daily routine. Also, think about how you can spend less time sitting and being inactive.

If you feel that you are already doing all that you can, speak with your doctor about what else you can do. He or she may also refer you to a physical activity health professional for advice.

SOME NOTES ABOUT BEING PHYSICALLY ACTIVE SAFELY

• If you become breathless or uncomfortable while doing any physical activity, slow down or stop. Discuss this with your doctor as soon as you can.

• If you have been prescribed angina-relieving medicine, carry it with you when you are being physically active and follow your doctor's advice for its use.

• Know the warning signs of heart attack. The warning signs vary and usually last for at least 10 minutes. You may experience more than one of these: tightness, fullness, pressure, heaviness or pain in one or more of your chest, shoulders, neck, arms, back or jaw you may also feel short of breath, nauseous, a cold sweat, dizzy or light-headed.

If you experience these heart attack warning signs, immediately stop what you are doing and rest. If you are with someone, tell them what you are experiencing.

TOO MANY REASONS NOT TO BE PHYSICALLY ACTIVE?

Apart from lack of time, other factors that can impact on your physical activity levels are:

• Your weight

• Feeling shy or embarrassed

• Not feeling 'sporty'

• Poor health

• Having some form of injury or disability.

If your health is poor or you have some form of injury or disability, seek advice from your doctor about suitable ways for you to be physically active. Your doctor may refer you to a physical activity health professional to give you more specific advice.

If your reasons for not being active are because you are embarrassed to be active, or your weight makes it difficult or you just don't feel sporty enough, always remember that a great form of physical activity is walking. Most people can walk and you can do this anywhere – even around your home.

Being physically active doesn't mean that you have to join a gym or play some form of sport. Doing these things is great, but if they don't suit you, you don't have to do them. It's most important that you find types of physical activity that you are comfortable to do.

COMPARISON OF ENERGY (KILOJOULES) USED THROUGH DIFFERENT PHYSICAL ACTIVITIES

Here are some examples of how you can make small but important changes to increase your physical activity levels. Remember, it's the small changes together that can make a big difference.

Also remember that these are just examples. The key is to think about what activities you do and how you can make improvements.

Sedentary	kJ burned	Active	kJ burned
Waiting for 30 minutes for home delivery of food	4	Cooking for 30 minutes	**105**
Using a lawn service	0	Gardening and mowing each for 30 minutes a week	**1505**
Letting the dog out the back door	8	Walking the dog for 30 minutes	**523**
Driving 40 minutes, walking five minutes (parking)	92	Walking 15 minutes to bus stop twice a day	**500**
Hiring someone to clean and iron	0	Ironing and vacuuming each for 30 minutes	**635**
Taking elevator or lift up three flights of stairs	1	Walking up three flights of stairs	**63**
Parking as close as possible, 10 second walk	1	Parking slightly further away, walking two minutes	**33**

Playing a computer game for 30 minutes	80	Playing a ball game for 30 minutes	546
Using the remote control to change TV channel	< 4	Getting up and changing the TV channel	13
Driving to the corner shop to get the paper	8	Walking to the corner shop for 10 minutes	167
Getting off the bus and walking five minutes to work	84	Getting off the bus one stop earlier and walking 15 minutes to work	252
Shopping online for one hour	125	Shopping at a mall, walking one hour	606–1003
Driving to local shops for lunch	8	Meeting a friend and walking 20 minutes to a local café	334
Reclining while talking on the phone for 30 minutes	16	Standing while talking on the phone for 30 minutes	84

CHAPTER SIX

STEP 5

KEEP GOING WITH YOUR WEIGHT LOSS PLAN

DECIDING WHAT CHANGES YOU CAN MAKE

After you've worked out where you think you could make some changes to what you eat and drink, your physical activity levels and sitting time, think about where you will start.

Although you might be keen to do it all at once, it's best to do things gradually. What you are trying to do may not be easy– you need to change your way of life and that's going to take some time, so give yourself time. Start with a change you think you can make fairly easily and give yourself a realistic amount of time to achieve it. Once you've managed one change, try the next one on your list.

Some examples of changes you might choose are:

• In the next fortnight, I will change to reduced fat milk instead of full cream milk

• I am going to go for a 15 minute walk on two evenings each week for the next month

• I'm going to eat two pieces of fruit each day this week

• Rather than use the escalator, I'm going to take the stairs instead

• I'm going to cut my TV viewing to one hour on three days this week.

REVIEW YOUR GOAL AND YOUR CHANGES

It's important to stop and reflect on how you are going with things. Have you achieved what you set out to do? If so, then give yourself a pat on the back and reward yourself.

If you haven't quite achieved what you wanted to, don't be discouraged. Now is the time to reflect on what you set out to do. Think about if you have:

• Tried to do too much too soon – remember, small changes over time are best

• Given yourself enough time – maybe you just need another month or two to make it happen

• Tried to do something that just isn't right for you – is there something else that you should try?

REWARD YOURSELF

Don't forget to spoil yourself every now and then. Changing your eating patterns, increasing your physical activity levels and losing weight is not that easy. So when you achieve a change, make sure you give yourself some sort of reward. Some examples are:

• Go to a movie

• Buy yourself something that you want, rather than need

• Go to a theatre show, a concert or a sporting event

• Go out to a nice restaurant for dinner

• Buy some new clothes

• Go on a nice outing with family or friends

• Buy yourself a new book to read

- Buy your favourite magazine

- Get some fresh flowers for your home

- Buy a nice pot plant at the market or local nursery

- Phone a friend overseas who you haven't spoken with for a while

- Buy some new sporting attire or equipment

- Buy a pedometer – a great motivational tool to track your physical activity

- Visit a place you enjoy – the beach, a park or a museum

- Visit friends

- Enjoy a weekend away

- Have a massage.

CHAPTER SEVEN

HEALTHY MEAL IDEAS

Don't worry if you have a day where you feel that it's all too hard or you haven't been able to keep up with your changes. We all have days like that. Just make sure that the changes you've set yourself suit you and then keep going with them.

Following are some ideas for healthier, lower energy (kilojoule) meals and snack options.

FOOD AT HOME

Breakfast Toast

• Use wholegrain or wholemeal bread.

• Try toppings such as a small serve of baked beans, tomatoes, creamed corn, mushrooms or cottage cheese.

• Spread toast thinly with jam, honey or peanut butter – these are all high in energy (kilojoules) so try to limit the amount you use.

• Use margarine spreads made from canola, sunflower or olive oil, or dairy blends.

• Breakfast cereals.

• Choose an untoasted, high fibre, wholegrain cereal, such as rolled oats, wheat biscuits or bran cereals.

• Use reduced, low or no fat milk, or 'added calcium' soy beverages.

• Add fruit – fresh, stewed or canned fruit (choose fruit canned in natural juice or unsweetened, or drain the liquid from the fruit).

• Add reduced, low or no fat yoghurt.

OTHER IDEAS

• Poach, boil or scramble eggs (use reduced, low or no fat milk). Serve with tomatoes, spinach, mushrooms and salmon or lean, reduced salt ham. Serve on wholegrain or whole meal bread.

• Make pancakes using reduced, low or no fat milk or buttermilk, whole meal flour and margarine spread made from canola, sunflower or olive oil, or dairy blends that have earned the Heart Foundation Tick instead of butter.

• Chop fresh fruit and top with reduced, low or no fat yoghurt.

SNACKS

• Snack on fruit – fresh, stewed or canned (choose fruit canned in natural juice or unsweetened, or drain the liquid from the fruit).

• Choose reduced, low or no fat yoghurt (plain or flavoured).

• Crunch on a small handful of plain, unsalted nuts.*

• Snack on wholegrain or wholemeal crisp bread with sliced tomato and pepper.

• Choose muesli bars with the Heart Foundation Tick.

• Enjoy a cup of vegetable soup (choose reduced salt).

*Nuts can contribute to an excess energy (kilojoule) intake so limit the quantity and frequency of eating them.

LUNCH SANDWICHES

• Fill sandwiches with lots of salad vegetables and a small serving of lean meat, skinless chicken, canned fish, hommus or a low fat cheese, such as cottage cheese.

• Make toasted sandwiches. Try fillings such as baked beans, lean meats, pineapple, tomatoes and vegetables, such as corn, spinach, asparagus and capsicum.

• Use wholemeal or wholegrain bread or rolls and margarine spreads made from canola, sunflower or olive oil, or dairy blends that have earned the Heart Foundation Tick instead of butter.

• Try different varieties of bread, e.g. focaccia, pita, bagels and mountain bread.

SALADS

• Include lots of different vegetables.

• Try adding fresh fruit or plain, unsalted nuts.

• Add legumes, such as four bean mix or chickpeas.

• Try pasta (preferably wholemeal), rice (preferably brown), couscous or noodle salads.

• Add lean meats, skinless poultry or fish.

• Use salad dressings and mayonnaise made from oils such as canola, sunflower, soybean and olive oil. Serve dressings and mayonnaise on the side so that people can add their own if they wish.

SOUPS

• Try vegetable- or legume-based soups. Serve with crusty bread to make a meal.

• Use evaporated skim milk instead of cream or full fat milk for 'creamy soups'.

OTHER IDEAS

• Make home-made pizza using a small pita bread (preferably wholemeal) as the base. Add reduced salt tomato paste, a small amount of reduced fat cheese, pineapple and vegetables, such as mushrooms, onion and capsicum.

• Rye crackers with tomato, basil and black pepper.

• Rice paper rolls or sushi.

• Tub of fruit salad with reduced, low or no fat yoghurt.

EVENING MEAL STIR-FRY DISHES

• Include lots of vegetables and use lean meat, skinless chicken or fish.

• Serve with pasta (preferably wholemeal), rice (preferably brown), couscous or noodles.

• Use oils such as canola, sunflower, soybean, olive, sesame and peanut oil.

• Add legumes, such as chickpeas, or some chopped plain, unsalted nuts, such as cashews or peanuts.*

• Flavour with herbs and spices, e.g. garlic, onion, chilli or ginger.

*Nuts can contribute to an excess energy (kilojoule) intake so limit the quantity and frequency of eating them.

PASTA DISHES

• Try wholemeal pasta varieties.

• Make a vegetable-based sauce, such as tomato or pumpkin.

• Add lean meats or fish and lots of vegetables.

• Use ricotta cheese or light evaporated skim milk to make a 'creamy' sauce instead of using cream.

• Use a small amount of reduced fat cheese or parmesan cheese.

• Serve with a garden salad.

MEAT AND VEGETABLES

• Use lean cuts of meat, skinless poultry or fish.

• Serve meat with vegetables or salad and a grain-based food, such as pasta (preferably wholemeal), rice (preferably brown), couscous or polenta.

• Use oils such as canola, sunflower, soybean, olive or peanut oil to cook meat and vegetables.

• Use herbs, spices and garlic to add flavour.

• Add reduced, low or no fat natural yoghurt to jacket potatoes instead of using sour cream.

• Roast meat on a rack in a roasting pan with a little water, wine or reduced salt stock.

• Brush or spray roast vegetables with oil such as canola, sunflower, soybean or olive oil and bake in a separate dish.

RICE OR NOODLE DISHES

• Try brown rice.

• Add lots of vegetables.

• Use lean meats, skinless poultry or fish.

• Use oils such as canola, sunflower, soybean, olive or peanut oil.

OTHER IDEAS

• Make burritos, tacos or tortilla wraps using lean meat, skinless chicken or red kidney beans. Add plenty of vegetables to the mixture and use reduced, low or no fat natural yoghurt instead of sour cream.

• Vegetable frittata or quiche. Use reduced, low or no fat milk and margarine spreads made from canola, sunflower or olive oil, or dairy blends that have earned the Heart Foundation Tick instead of butter to make the quiche. Serve with a garden salad.

• Make a pie using filo pastry for the top and bottom or only have a pastry lid. Use lean meat, skinless chicken or fish and lots of vegetables for the filling.

BARBECUES

• Trim all visible fat from meat before cooking.

• Marinate skinless chicken breast fillets, fish, seafood or lean meat in fruit juice or wine and herbs before cooking on the barbecue.

• Bake fish fillets in foil with seasonings and lemon juice.

• Make kebabs using lean meat and/or vegetable chunks.

• Slice vegetables, such as mushrooms, eggplant, sweet potato and zucchini, and cook on the barbecue.

• Use margarine spreads made from canola, sunflower or olive oil, or dairy blends that have earned the Heart Foundation Tick instead of butter. Use oils such as canola, sunflower, soybean, olive or peanut oil.

• Serve wholegrain or whole meal bread.

• Serve a variety of salads. Use salad dressings and mayonnaise made from oils such as canola, sunflower, soybean and olive oils. Serve dressings and mayonnaise on the side so that people can add their own if they wish.

DESSERTS

• Fresh fruit salad, stewed, poached or canned fruit served with reduced, low or no fat yoghurt. Choose fruit canned in natural juice or unsweetened, or drain the liquid from the fruit.

• Fruit-based puddings or crumbles made with margarine spread, wholemeal flour, oats and reduced, low or no fat milk. Use margarine spreads made from canola, sunflower or olive oil, or dairy blends that have earned the Heart Foundation Tick instead of butter.

• Fruit pie or strudel made with filo pastry. Serve with reduced, low or no fat yoghurt.

• Cheesecake made using reduced fat cream cheese or ricotta cheese, margarine spread and plain sweet biscuits. Use margarine spreads made from canola, sunflower or olive oil, or dairy blends. Add lots of fruit on top or add fruit into the cheese mixture.

• Low fat ice-cream or diet jelly. Serve with fruit.

TAKE-AWAY FOODS

Take-away food is quick and convenient, but it can be a real trap if you're trying to lose weight. Many take-away foods are high in energy (kilojoules), so choose carefully.

• Try to limit pastries (such as pies or pasties), pizza, hamburgers, hot chips, fried fish, fried chicken and creamy pasta dishes to no more than once a week. Instead choose take-away foods that contain lots of vegetables. Some suggestions follow.

ASIAN MEALS

• Healthier choices include steamed rice, mixed vegetable dishes, lean meats (beef, lamb, pork or chicken), fish, seafood and stir-fries.

• Try to limit deep-fried menu options.

ITALIAN MEALS

• Choose pasta dishes with vegetable-based sauces.

• Choose thin crust pizza with pineapple, tomato and lots of vegetables, such as onion, capsicum, mushrooms, artichoke, eggplant and pumpkin. Try to avoid pizzas with salami or sausage meats. Instead, ask for lean meats, such as fish or lean reduced salt ham. Ask for a small amount of cheese or for reduced fat cheese.

GREEK/LEBANESE MEALS

• Choose souvlaki/shish kebabs in pita bread with tabouli or Lebanese bread with salad.

• Choose stuffed vegetable dishes.

• Limit pastries.

BARBECUE CHICKEN

• Choose the breast meat – chicken breast has a lower fat content. Remove the skin and fat and limit gravy and stuffing. The breadcrumbs and flour in the stuffing tend to soak up a lot of fat and the gravy is generally high in fat and salt.

• Grab some salad or vegetable dishes to have with the chicken rather than chips.

• Hamburgers/Steak sandwiches

• If they're made with lean grilled meat and lots of salad, hamburgers/ steak sandwiches can make a nutritious meal without too much energy (kilojoules). Where possible, ask for extra salad and a wholegrain or wholemeal bun or bread.

SANDWICHES AND BREAD ROLLS

• Ask for sandwiches and bread rolls to be made with margarine spreads made from canola, sunflower or olive oil, or dairy blends that have earned the Heart Foundation Tick instead of butter, and fillings such as lean meat, low or reduced fat cheese, skinless chicken, salmon, tuna or felafel, and plenty of salad vegetables. Ask for wholegrain or wholemeal bread.

CORN ON THE COB

• Choose plain corn on the cob, rather than with butter.

JACKET POTATOES

• Choose beans and salads as the main toppings and some margarine spreads made from canola, sunflower or olive oil, or dairy blends that have earned the Heart Foundation Tick instead of butter. Ask for a small amount of cheese or a reduced fat cheese, and for reduced, low or no fat natural yoghurt instead of sour cream.

SALAD BARS

• These usually offer a range of choices. Some types of salad, such as bean salad and pasta salad, can make a complete meal on their own. The main thing to watch for is the dressings and mayonnaise used – these are often high in saturated fat. Where possible, choose salads with a dressing or mayonnaise made from oils such as canola, sunflower, soybean or olive oil, or choose salads without dressings or with the dressing on the side.

EATING OUT

• Always read the menu carefully and don't be afraid to ask questions of the staff to help you to make your decision. Most cafés and restaurants will be more than happy to help and will do their best to provide you with a suitable meal. Some food outlets even provide nutritional information about their dishes.

SOME TIPS

• Choose a meal with vegetables, legumes or salad included, or order these as a side dish.

• Ask for your vegetables to be served lightly steamed or microwaved, without added sauce or butter.

• Ask for your meal to be served without chips.

• Ask for salad dressing and mayonnaise made from oils such as canola, sunflower, soybean and olive oil, and ask for this on the side so you can add it yourself.

• Ask about ingredients or sauces – if they contain butter or cream, ask for them not to be added to your meal.

• Choose seafood dishes that aren't crumbed or fried.

• Choose pasta dishes with a vegetable-based sauce instead of a creamy one. Also try to limit sauces with fatty meats, such as bacon and sausage.

• Choose dishes containing lean meats. If you are served meat with fat, then remove it before eating. For example, remove the skin and fat from poultry, and trim fat from meat.

• Ask for smaller meals – perhaps a half serve if it's an option, or choose an entrée-sized dish.

• If you're eating in an outlet that offers larger serves at a cheaper price, try not to choose this option. It may be value for money, but it's not value for your health.

• 'All you can eat' and smorgasbords can encourage you to eat much more than you need. Try not to pile food onto your plate or go back for seconds. If there are lots of dishes you'd love to try, just have a small serving of the most appealing ones. You can always visit another time and try the dishes you've missed out on this time. If you really want to limit the amount of food you're eating, then use a smaller plate.

• Ask for plain, fresh bread (preferably wholegrain or wholemeal) instead of garlic and herb breads. Garlic and herb breads are high in energy (kilojoules).

DESSERTS

• Choose fruit-based options, such as baked fruit, poached fruit or fresh fruit salad. Ask for some reduced, low or no fat yoghurt or a small serve of low or reduced fat ice-cream.

• Suggest sharing a dessert with someone else at your table – that way you get to enjoy a treat, but the energy (kilojoules) is shared.

• Choose sorbets.

CONCLUSION

We always want to look good and to feel good. When we grow up and become adults, we get more conscious on how we look like. We try different types of dieting methods. We follow fads and trends here and there. We compete with our friends and colleagues and even to ourselves just to get the right body we want. We see everything on TV, we hear the news about how people lose weight and we encounter these weight loss products. Most of them do not really work. While everyone still struggles on the process of dieting, this article has already given the basic secrets to successful lose weight dieting. Some people may already have started but for those who are still on the verge of deciding whether to try it out, be confident that you will get better results. It is recommended that you not only eat good food but you enjoy them at the same time. We also emphasize that you should learn the habit of eating delicious food as it becomes easier to lose weight.

Weight control methods can be successful if lose weight dieting is maintained without compromising overall health. When you get successful in weight reduction program, you also promote permanent life-style changes. The physical and psychological benefits of maintaining the right weight can be observed when it is done are the right way. It is, however, more beneficial when you personalize the weight reduction plan based on individual's needs and lifestyle.

When you get the right ingredients of lose weight dieting like exercise and sleep, you tend to get the weight you desire. We know that getting the right weight also prevents us from certain diseases. Not only that, we function well in our daily workload. We become successful when we do our job right.

For all of us, it is definitely important that we look good. By getting the proper nutrition and understanding how the body works, we get the optimum level of health and it gives you the glow you deserve. Sometimes, we just overlooked the secrets of getting the best of us. We miss to identify how we get through with getting healthy and looking good. Therefore, being conscious about our weight and our physical appearance is not bad at all. It actually reflects on how we live our lives and how we become effective creatures. Being healthy gives you an overall functionality.

ABOUT THE AUTHOR

Jessica Mace is a nutritional therapist and researcher who has done a lot of work in preventing and reversing excessive weight gain. She has an effective and engaging approach to weight loss and her methods have been helping a lot of people.

She is married and lives with her husband and 2 children.